C000081985

Special Plant-Based Recipes Collection

Stay Healthy with These Tasty Recipes

Lily Mullen

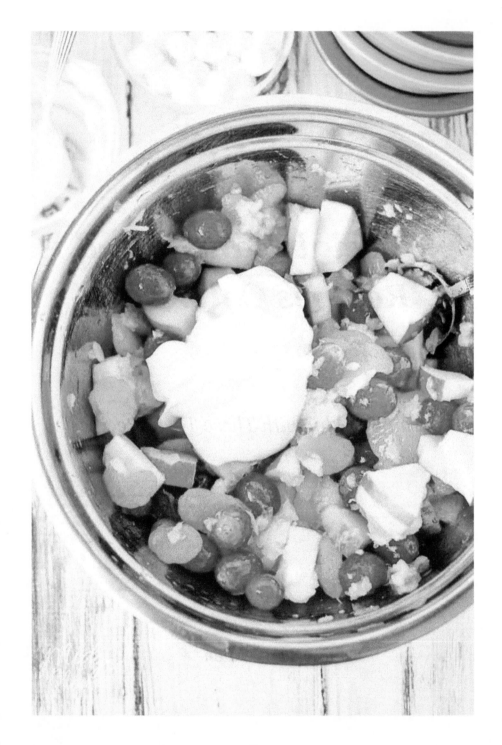

TABLE OF CONTENTS

Introduction

A plant-based eating routine backing and upgrades the entirety of this. For what reason should most of what we eat originate from the beginning?

Eating more plants is the first nourishing convention known to man to counteract and even turn around the ceaseless diseases that assault our general public.

Plants and vegetables are brimming with large scale and micronutrients that give our bodies all that we require for a sound and productive life. By eating, at any rate, two suppers stuffed with veggies consistently, and nibbling on foods grown from the ground in the middle of, the nature of your wellbeing and at last your life will improve.

The most widely recognized wellbeing worries that individuals have can be reduced by this one straightforward advance.

Things like weight, inadequate rest, awful skin, quickened maturing, irritation, physical torment, and absence of vitality would all be able to be decidedly influenced by expanding the admission of plants and characteristic nourishments.

If you're reading this book, then you're probably on a journey to get healthy because you know good health and nutrition go hand in hand.

Maybe you're looking at the plant-based diet as a solution to those love handles.

Whatever the case may be, the standard American diet millions of people eat daily is not the best way to fuel your body.

If you ask me, any other diet will already be a significant improvement. Since what you eat fuels your body, you can imagine that eating junk will make you feel just that—like junk.

I've followed the standard American diet for several years: my plate was loaded with high-fat and carbohydrate-rich foods. I know this doesn't sound like a horrible way to eat, but keep in mind that most Americans don't focus on eating healthy fats and complex carbs—we live on processed foods.

The consequences of eating foods filled with trans fats, preservatives, and mountains of sugar are fatigue, reduced mental focus, mood swings, and weight gain. To top it off, there's the issue of opening yourself up to certain diseases— some life-threatening—when you neglect paying attention to what you eat .

Lentil and Chickpea Salad

Preparation time: 10 minutes

Cooking time: 0 minute

Servings: 4

Ingredients:

For the Lemon Dressing:

- ¼ cup lemon juice
- 2 tablespoons olive oil
- 1 teaspoon Dijon mustard
- 1 teaspoon honey or maple syrup
- ½ teaspoon minced garlic
- ¼ teaspoon of sea salt
- ¼ teaspoon ground black pepper

For the Salad:

- 2 cups French green lentils, cooked
- 1 ½ cups cooked chickpeas
- 1 medium avocado, pitted, sliced
- 1 big bunch of radishes, chopped
- ¼ cup chopped mint and dill

- Crumbled vegan feta cheese as needed

Directions:

1. Prepare the dressing and for this, place all of its ingredients in a bowl and whisk until combined.
2. Take a large bowl, place all the ingredients for the salad in it, drizzle with the dressing and toss until combined.
3. Serve straight away.

Roasted Carrots with Farro, and Chickpeas

Preparation time: 10 minutes

Cooking time: 35 minutes

Servings: 4

Ingredients:

For the Chickpeas and Farro:

- 1 cup farro, cooked
- 1 ½ cups cooked chickpeas
- ½ teaspoon minced garlic
- 1 teaspoon lemon juice
- ½ teaspoon salt
- 1 teaspoon olive oil

For the Roasted Carrots:

- 1 pound heirloom carrots, scrubbed
- ½ teaspoon ground black pepper
- ¼ teaspoon ground cumin
- 1 teaspoon salt
- 1 tablespoon olive oil

For the Spiced Pepitas:

- 3 tablespoons green pumpkin seeds
- 1/8 teaspoon salt
- 1/8 teaspoon red chili powder
- 1/8 teaspoon cumin
- ½ teaspoon olive oil

For the Crème Fraiche:

- 1 tablespoon chopped parsley
- 1/3 cup vegan crème fraîche
- ¼ teaspoon ground black pepper
- 1/3 teaspoon salt
- 2 teaspoons water

For the Garnish:

- 1 more tablespoon chopped parsley

Directions:

1. Prepare chickpeas and farro and for this, place all of its ingredients in a bowl and toss until combined.
2. Prepare the carrots and for this, arrange them on a baking sheet lined with parchment paper, drizzle with oil, sprinkle with the seasoning, toss until coated, and bake for 35 minutes until roasted and fork-tender, turning halfway.

3. Meanwhile, prepare pepitas and for this, take a skillet pan, place it over medium heat, add oil and when hot, add remaining ingredients in it and cook for 3 minutes until seeds are golden on the edges, set aside, and let it cool.

4. Prepare the crème Fraiche and for this, place all its ingredients in a bowl and whisk until combined.

5. Top chickpeas and farro with carrots, drizzle with crème Fraiche, sprinkle with pepitas and parsley and then serve.

Spaghetti Squash Burrito Bowls

Preparation time: 10 minutes

Cooking time: 60 minutes

Servings: 4

Ingredients:

For the Spaghetti Squash:

- 2 medium spaghetti squash , halved, deseeded
- 2 tablespoons olive oil
- 1 teaspoon salt
- ½ teaspoon ground black pepper

For the Slaw:

- 1/3 cup chopped green onions
- 2 cups chopped purple cabbage
- 1/3 cup chopped cilantro
- 15 ounces cooked black beans
- 1 medium red bell pepper, cored, chopped
- ¼ teaspoon salt
- 1 teaspoon olive oil
- 2 tablespoons lime juice

For the Salsa Verde:

- 1 avocado, pitted, diced
- ½ teaspoon minced garlic
- ¾ cup salsa verde
- 1/3 cup cilantro
- 1 tablespoon lime juice

Directions:

1. Prepare the squash and for this, place squash halves on a baking sheet lined with parchment paper, rub them with oil, season with salt and black pepper and bake for 60 minutes until roasted and fork-tender.
2. Meanwhile, place the slaw and for this, place all of its ingredients in a bowl and toss until combined.
3. Prepare the salsa, and for this, place all of its ingredients in a food processor and pulse until smooth.
4. When squash has baked, fluff its flesh with a fork, then top with slaw and salsa and serve.

Spanish Rice

Preparation time: 5 minutes

Cooking time: 40 minutes

Servings: 4

Ingredients:

- 1/2 of medium green bell pepper, chopped
- 1 medium white onion, peeled, chopped
- 10 ounces diced tomatoes with green chilies
- 1 teaspoon salt
- 2 teaspoons red chili powder
- 1 cup white rice
- 2 tablespoons olive oil
- 2 cups of water

Directions:

1. Take a large skillet pan, place it over medium heat, add oil and when hot, add onion, pepper, and rice, and cook for 10 minutes.
2. Then add remaining ingredients, stir until mixed, bring the mixture to a boil, then simmer over medium-low heat

for 30 minutes until cooked and most of the liquid has absorbed.

3. Serve straight away.

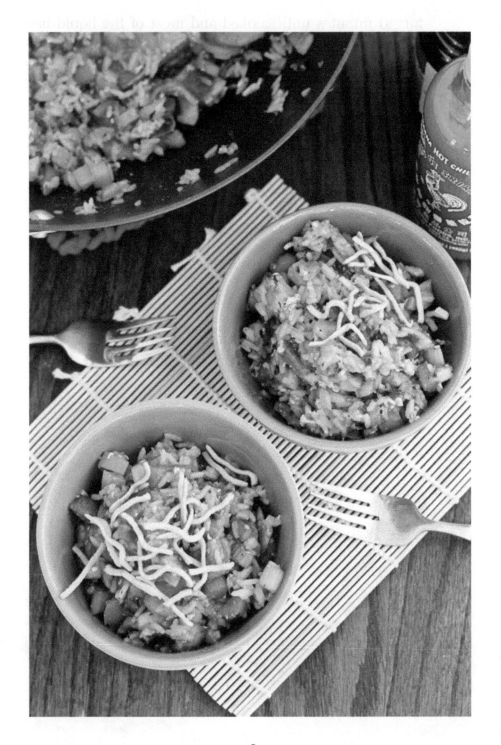

Black Beans and Rice

Preparation time: 10 minutes

Cooking time: 30 minutes

Servings: 4

Ingredients:

- 3/4 cup white rice
- 1 medium white onion, peeled, chopped
- 3 1/2 cups cooked black beans
- 1 teaspoon minced garlic
- 1/4 teaspoon cayenne pepper
- 1 teaspoon ground cumin
- 1 teaspoon olive oil
- 1 1/2 cups vegetable broth

Directions:

1. Take a large pot over medium-high heat, add oil and when hot, add onion and garlic and cook for 4 minutes until saute.

2. Then stir in rice, cook for 2 minutes, pour in the broth, bring it to a boil, switch heat to the low level and cook for 20 minutes until tender.

3. Stir in remaining ingredients, cook for 2 minutes, and then serve straight away.

Lentils and Rice with Fried Onions

Preparation time: 5 minutes

Cooking time: 7 minutes

Servings: 4

Ingredients:

- 3/4 cup long-grain white rice, cooked
- 1 large white onion, peeled, sliced
- 1 1/3 cups green lentils, cooked
- ½ teaspoon salt
- 1/4 cup vegan sour cream
- ¼ teaspoon ground black pepper
- 6 tablespoons olive oil

Directions:

1. Take a large skillet pan, place it over medium heat, add oil and when hot, add onions, and cook for 10 minutes until browned, set aside until required.

2. Take a saucepan, place it over medium heat, grease it with oil, add lentils and beans and cook for 3 minutes until warmed.

3. Season with salt and black pepper, cook for 2 minutes, then stir in half of the browned onions, and top with cream and remaining onions.

4. Serve straight away.

Mexican Stuffed Peppers

Preparation time: 10 minutes

Cooking time: 40 minutes

Servings: 4

Ingredients:

- 2 cups cooked rice
- 1/2 cup chopped onion
- 15 ounces cooked black beans
- 4 large green bell peppers, destemmed, cored
- 1 tablespoon olive oil
- 1 tablespoon salt
- 14.5 ounce diced tomatoes
- 1/2 teaspoon ground cumin
- 1 teaspoon garlic salt
- 1 teaspoon red chili powder
- 1/2 teaspoon salt
- 2 cups shredded vegan
- Mexican cheese blend

Directions:

1. Boil the bell peppers in salty water for 5 minutes until softened and then set aside until required.

2. Heat oil over medium heat in a skillet pan, then add onion and cook for 10 minutes until softened.

3. Transfer the onion mixture in a bowl, add remaining ingredients, reserving ½ cup cheese blended, stir until mixed, and then fill this mixture into the boiled peppers.

4. Arrange the peppers in the square baking dish, sprinkle them with remaining cheese and bake for 30 minutes at 350 degrees F.

5. Serve straight away.

Mushroom Risotto

Preparation time: 10 minutes

Cooking time: 35 minutes

Servings: 4

Ingredients:

- 1 cup of rice
- 3 small white onions, peeled, chopped
- 1 teaspoon minced celery
- 1 ½ cups sliced mushrooms
- ½ teaspoon minced garlic
- 1 teaspoon minced parsley
- ½ teaspoon salt
- ¼ teaspoon ground black pepper
- 1 tablespoon olive oil
- 1 teaspoon vegan butter
- ¼ cup vegan cashew cream
- 1 cup grated vegan Parmesan cheese
- 1 cup of coconut milk
- 5 cups vegetable stock

Directions:

1. Take a large skillet pan, place it over medium-high heat, add oil and when hot, add onion and garlic, and cook for 5 minutes.
2. Transfer to a plate, add celery and parsley into the pan, stir in salt and black pepper, and cook for 3 minutes.
3. Then switch heat to medium-low level, stir in mushrooms, cook for 5 minutes, then pour in cream and milk, stir in rice until combined, and bring the mixture to simmer.
4. Pour in vegetable stock, one cup at a time until it has absorbed and, when done, stir in cheese and butter.
5. Serve straight away.

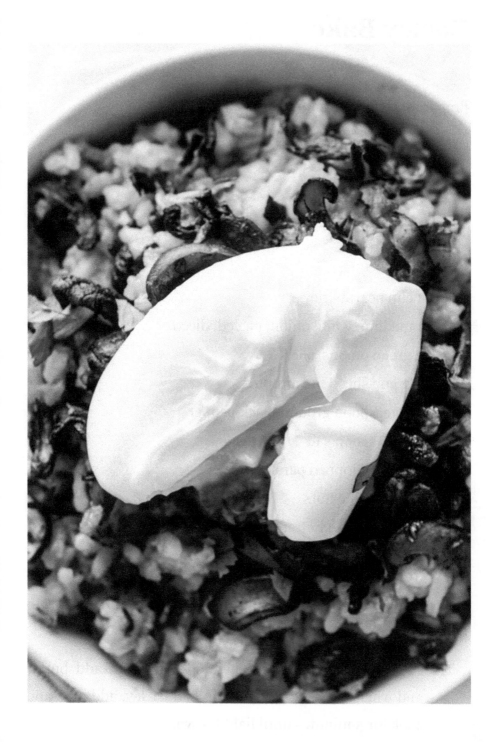

Barley Bake

Preparation time: 10 minutes

Cooking time: 98 minutes

Servings: 6

Ingredients:

- 1 cup pearl barley
- 1 medium white onion, peeled, diced
- 2 green onions, sliced
- 1/2 cup sliced mushrooms
- 1/8 teaspoon ground black pepper
- 1/4 teaspoon salt
- 1/2 cup chopped parsley
- 1/2 cup pine nuts
- 1/4 cup vegan butter
- 29 ounces vegetable broth

Directions:

1. Place a skillet pan over medium-high heat, add butter and when it melts, stir in onion and barley, add nuts and cook for 5 minutes until light brown.

2. Add mushrooms, green onions and parsley, sprinkle with salt and black pepper, cook for 1 minute and then transfer the mixture into a casserole dish.
3. Pour in broth, stir until mixed and bake for 90 minutes until barley is tender and has absorbed all the liquid.
4. Serve straight away

Mushroom, Lentil, and Barley Stew

Preparation time: 10 minutes

Cooking time: 6 hours Servings: 8

Ingredients:

- 3/4 cup pearl barley
- 2 cups sliced button mushrooms
- 3/4 cup dry lentils
- 1 ounce dried shiitake mushrooms
- 2 teaspoons minced garlic
- 1/4 cup dried onion flakes
- 2 teaspoons ground black pepper
- 1 teaspoon dried basil
- 2 ½ teaspoons salt
- 2 teaspoons dried savory
- 3 bay leaves
- 2 quarts vegetable broth

Directions:

1. Switch on the slow cooker, place all the ingredients in it, and stir until combined.
2. Shut with lid and cook the stew for 6 hours at a high heat setting until cooked.
3. Serve straight away.

Black Beans, Corn, and Yellow Rice

Preparation time: 10 minutes

Cooking time: 25 minutes

Servings: 8

Ingredients:

- 8 ounces yellow rice mix
- 15.25 ounces cooked kernel corn
- 1 1/4 cups water
- 15 ounces cooked black beans
- 1 teaspoon ground cumin
- 2 teaspoons lime juice
- 2 tablespoons olive oil

Directions:

1. Place a saucepan over high heat, add oil, water, and rice, bring the mixture to a bowl, and then switch heat to medium-low level.

2. Simmer for 25 minutes until rice is tender and all the liquid has been absorbed and then transfer the rice to a large bowl.

3. Add remaining ingredients into the rice, stir until mixed and serve straight away

Cuban Beans and Rice

Preparation time: 10 minutes

Cooking time: 55 minutes

Servings: 6

Ingredients:

- 1 cup uncooked white rice
- 1 green bell pepper, cored, chopped
- 15.25 ounces cooked kidney beans
- 1 cup chopped white onion
- 4 tablespoons tomato paste
- 1 teaspoon minced garlic
- 1 teaspoon salt
- 1 tablespoon olive oil
- 2 ½ cups vegetable broth

Directions:

1. Take a saucepan, place it over medium heat, add oil and when hot, add onion, garlic and bell pepper and cook for 5 minutes until tender.

2. Then stir in salt and tomatoes, switch heat to the low level and cook for 2 minutes.

3. Then stir in rice and beans, pour in the broth, stir until mixed and cook for 45 minutes until rice has absorbed all the liquid.

4. Serve straight away.

Pecan Rice

Preparation time: 5 minutes

Cooking time: 10 minutes

Servings: 4

Ingredients:

- 1/4 cup chopped white onion
- 1/4 teaspoon ground ginger
- 1/2 cup chopped pecans
- 1/4 teaspoon salt
- 2 tablespoons minced parsley
- 1/4 teaspoon ground black pepper
- 1/4 teaspoon dried basil
- 2 tablespoons vegan margarine
- 1 cup brown rice, cooked

Directions:

1. Take a skillet pan, place it over medium heat, add margarine and when it melts, add all the ingredients except for rice and stir until mixed.

2. Cook for 5 minutes, then stir in rice until combined and continue cooking for 2 minutes.
3. Serve straight away

Lentil, Rice and Vegetable Bake

Preparation time: 10 minutes

Cooking time: 40 minutes

Servings: 6

Ingredients:

- 1/2 cup white rice, cooked
- 1 cup red lentils, cooked
- 1/3 cup chopped carrots
- 1 medium tomato, chopped
- 1 small onion, peeled, chopped
- 1/3 cup chopped zucchini
- 1/3 cup chopped celery
- 1 ½ teaspoon minced garlic
- ½ teaspoon ground black pepper
- 1 teaspoon dried basil
- 1 teaspoon ground cumin
- 1 teaspoon dried oregano
- ½ teaspoon salt
- 1 teaspoon olive oil
- 8 ounces tomato sauce

Directions:

1. Take a skillet pan, place it over medium heat, add oil and when hot, add onion and garlic, and cook for 5 minutes.
2. Then add remaining vegetables, season with salt, black pepper, and half of each cumin, oregano and basil and cook for 5 minutes until vegetables are tender.
3. Take a casserole dish, place lentils and rice in it, top with vegetables, spread with tomato sauce and sprinkle with remaining cumin, oregano, and basil, and bake for 30 minutes until bubbly.
4. Serve straight away

Quinoa and Chickpeas Salad

Preparation time: 10 minutes

Cooking time: 0 minute

Servings: 4

Ingredients:

- 3/4 cup chopped broccoli
- 1/2 cup quinoa, cooked
- 15 ounces cooked chickpeas
- ½ teaspoon minced garlic
- 1/3 teaspoon ground black pepper
- 2/3 teaspoon salt
- 1 teaspoon dried tarragon
- 2 teaspoons mustard
- 1 tablespoon lemon juice
- 3 tablespoons olive oil

Directions:

1. Take a large bowl, place all the ingredients in it, and stir until well combined.
2. Serve straight away.

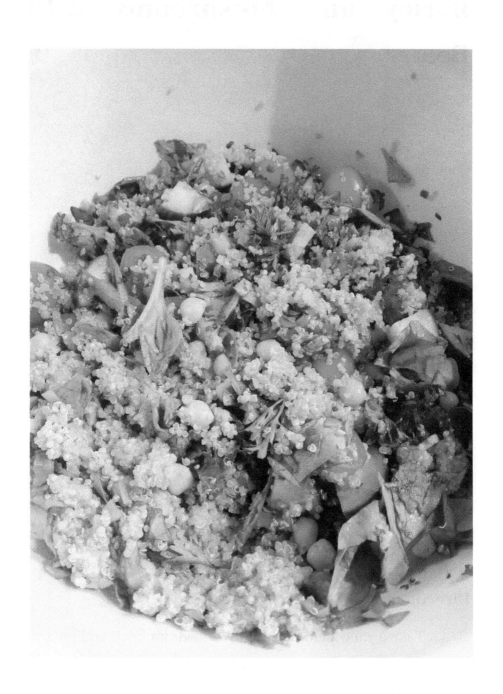

Barley and Mushrooms with Beans

Preparation time: 5 minutes

Cooking time: 15 minutes

Servings: 6

Ingredients:

- 1/2 cup uncooked barley
- 15.5 ounces white beans
- 1/2 cup chopped celery
- 3 cups sliced mushrooms
- 1 cup chopped white onion
- 1 teaspoon minced garlic
- 1 teaspoon olive oil
- 3 cups vegetable broth

Directions:

1. Take a saucepan, place it over medium heat, add oil and when hot, add vegetables and cook for 5 minutes until tender.

2. Pour in broth, stir in barley, bring the mixture to boil, and then simmer for 50 minutes until tender.

3. When done, add beans into the barley mixture, stir until mixed and continue cooking for 5 minutes until hot.

4. Serve straight away.

Garlic and White Bean Soup

Cooking time: 10 minutes

Servings: 4

Ingredients:

- 45 ounces cooked cannellini beans
- 1/4 teaspoon dried thyme
- 2 teaspoons minced garlic
- 1/8 teaspoon crushed red pepper
- 1/2 teaspoon dried rosemary
- 1/8 teaspoon ground black pepper
- 2 tablespoons olive oil
- 4 cups vegetable broth

Directions:

1. Place one-third of white beans in a food processor, then pour in 2 cups broth and pulse for 2 minutes until smooth.
2. Place a pot over medium heat, add oil and when hot, add garlic and cook for 1 minute until fragrant.

3. Add pureed beans into the pan along with remaining beans, sprinkle with spices and herbs, pour in the broth, stir until combined, and bring the mixture to boil over medium-high heat.

4. Switch heat to medium-low level, simmer the beans for 15 minutes, and then mash them with a fork.

5. Taste the soup to adjust seasoning and then serve.

Tomato, Kale, and White Bean Skillet

Preparation time: 10 minutes

Cooking time: 10 minutes

Servings: 4

Ingredients:

- 30 ounces cooked cannellini beans
- 3.5 ounces sun-dried tomatoes, packed in oil, chopped
- 6 ounces kale, chopped
- 1 teaspoon minced garlic
- 1/4 teaspoon ground black pepper
- 1/4 teaspoon salt
- 1/2 tablespoon dried basil
- 1/8 teaspoon red pepper flakes
- 1 tablespoon apple cider vinegar
- 1 tablespoon olive oil
- 2 tablespoons oil from sun-dried tomatoes

Directions:

1. Prepare the dressing and for this, place basil, black pepper, salt, vinegar, and red pepper flakes in a small bowl, add oil from sun-dried tomatoes and whisk until combined.

2. Take a skillet pan, place it over medium heat, add olive oil and when hot, add garlic and cook for 1 minute until fragrant.

3. Add kale, splash with some water and cook for 3 minutes until kale leaves have wilted.

4. Add tomatoes and beans, stir well and cook for 3 minutes until heated.

5. Remove pan from heat, drizzle with the prepared dressing, toss until mixed and serve.

Quinoa Meatballs

Preparation time: 10 minutes

Cooking time: 35 minutes

Servings: 4

Ingredients:

- 1 cup quinoa, cooked
- 1 tablespoon flax meal
- 1 cup diced white onion
- 1 ½ teaspoon minced garlic
- 1/2 teaspoon salt
- 1 teaspoon dried oregano
- 1 teaspoon lemon zest
- 1 teaspoon paprika
- 1 teaspoon dried basil
- 3 tablespoons water
- 2 tablespoons olive oil
- 1 cup grated vegan mozzarella cheese
- Marinara sauce as needed for serving

Directions:

1. Place flax meal in a bowl, stir in water and set aside until required.

2. Take a large skillet pan, place it over medium heat, add 1 tablespoon oil and when hot, add onion and cook for 2 minutes.

3. Stir in all the spices and herbs, then stir in quinoa until combined and cook for 2 minutes.

4. Transfer quinoa mixture in a bowl, add flax meal mixture, lemon zest, and cheese, stir until well mixed and then shape the mixture into twelve 1 ½ inch balls.

5. Arrange balls on a baking sheet lined with parchment paper, refrigerate the balls for 30 minutes and then bake for 20 minutes at 400 degrees F.

6. Serve balls with marinara sauce

Pineapple Fried Rice

Preparation time: 5 minutes

Cooking time: 12 minutes

Servings: 2

Ingredients:

- 2 cups brown rice, cooked
- 1/2 cup sunflower seeds, toasted
- 2/3 cup green peas
- 1 teaspoon minced garlic
- 1 large red bell pepper, cored, diced
- 1 tablespoon grated ginger
- 2/3 cup pineapple chunks with juice
- 2 tablespoons coconut oil
- 1 bunch of green onions, sliced

For the Sauce:

- 4 tablespoons soy sauce
- 1/2 cup pineapple juice
- 1/2 teaspoon sesame oil
- 1/2 a lime, juiced

Directions:

1. Take a skillet pan, place it over medium-high heat, add oil and when hot, add red bell pepper, pineapple pieces, and two-third of onion, cook for 5 minutes, then stir in ginger and garlic and cook for 1 minute.

2. Switch heat to the high level, add rice to the pan, stir until combined and cook for 5 minutes.

3. When done, fold in sunflower seeds and peas and set aside until required.

4. Prepare the sauce and for this, place sesame oil in a small bowl, add soy sauce and pineapple juice and whisk until combined.

5. Drizzle sauce over rice, drizzle with lime juice, and serve straight away.

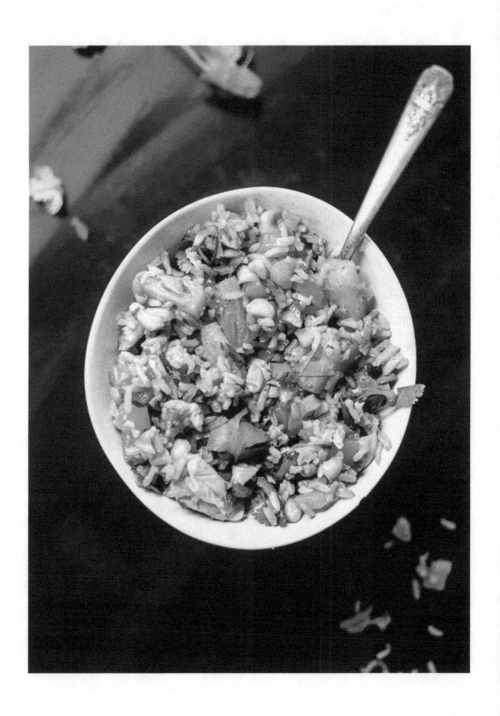

Black Bean Meatball Salad

Preparation time: 10 minutes

Cooking time: 25 minutes

Servings: 4

Ingredients:

For the Meatballs:

- 1/2 cup quinoa, cooked
- 1 cup cooked black beans
- 3 cloves of garlic, peeled
- 1 small red onion, peeled
- 1 teaspoon ground dried coriander
- 1 teaspoon ground dried cumin
- 1 teaspoon smoked paprika

For the Salad:

- 1 large sweet potato, peeled, diced
- 1 lemon, juiced
- 1 teaspoon minced garlic
- 1 cup coriander leaves
- 1/3 cup almonds

- 1/3 teaspoon ground black pepper
- ½ teaspoon salt
- 1 1/2 tablespoons olive oil

Directions:

1. Prepare the meatballs and for this, place beans and puree in a blender, pulse until pureed, and this place this mixture in a medium bowl.
2. Add onion and garlic, process until chopped, add to the bean mixture, add all the spices, stir until combined, and shape the mixture into uniform balls.
3. Bake the balls on a greased baking sheet for 25 minutes at 350 degrees F until browned.
4. Meanwhile, spread sweet potatoes on a baking sheet lined with baking paper, drizzle with ½ tablespoon oil, toss until coated and bake for 20 minutes with the meatballs.
5. Prepare the dressing, and for this, place remaining ingredients for the salad in a food processor and pulse until smooth.
6. Place roasted sweet potatoes in a bowl, drizzle with the dressing, toss until coated, and then top with meatballs.
7. Serve straight away.

Black Bean Stuffed Sweet Potatoes

Preparation time: 15 minutes

Cooking time: 65 minutes

Servings: 4

Ingredients:

- 4 large sweet potatoes
- 15 ounces cooked black beans
- 1/2 teaspoon ground black pepper
- 1/2 of a medium red onion, peeled, diced
- 1/2 teaspoon sea salt
- 1/4 teaspoon onion powder
- 1/4 teaspoon garlic powder
- 1/4 teaspoon red chili powder
- 1/4 teaspoon cumin
- 1 teaspoon lime juice
- 1 1/2 tablespoons olive oil
- 1/2 cup cashew cream sauce

Directions:

1. Spread sweet potatoes on a baking tray greased with oil and bake for 65 minutes at 350 degrees F until tender.

2. Meanwhile, prepare the sauce, and for this, whisk together the cream sauce, black pepper and lime juice until combined, set aside until required.

3. When 10 minutes of the baking time of potatoes are left, heat a skillet pan with oil, then add onion and cook for 5 minutes until golden.

4. Then stir in spice, cook for another 3 minutes, stir in bean until combined and cook for 5 minutes until hot.

5. Let roasted sweet potatoes cool for 10 minutes, then cut them open, mash the flesh and top with bean mixture, cilantro and avocado, and then drizzle with cream sauce.

6. Serve straight away.

Chickpea Fajitas

Preparation time: 10 minutes

Cooking time: 30 minutes

Servings: 4

Ingredients:

For the Chickpea Fajitas:

- 1 1/2 cups cooked chickpeas
- 1 medium white onion, peeled, sliced
- 2 medium green bell peppers, cored, sliced
- 1 tablespoon fajita seasoning
- 2 tablespoons olive oil

For the Cream:

- 1/2 cup cashews, soaked
- 1 clove of garlic, peeled
- ½ teaspoon salt
- 1/2 teaspoon ground cumin
- 1/4 cup lime juice
- 1/4 cup water
- 1 tablespoon olive oil

To serve:

- Sliced avocado for topping
- Chopped lettuce for topping
- 4 flour tortillas
- Chopped tomatoes for topping
- Salsa for topping
- Chopped cilantro for topping

Directions:

1. Prepare chickpeas and for this, whisk together seasoning and oil until combined, add onion, pepper, and chickpeas, toss until well coated, then spread them in a baking sheet and roast for 30 minutes at 400 degrees F until crispy and browned, stirring halfway.

2. Meanwhile, prepare the cream and for this, place all of its ingredients in a food processor and pulse until smooth, set aside until required.

3. When chickpeas and vegetables have roasted, top them evenly on tortillas, then top them evenly with avocado, lettuce, tomatoes, salsa, and cilantro and serve.

Mediterranean Chickpea Casserole

Preparation time: 10 minutes

Cooking time: 60 minutes

Servings: 4

Ingredients:

- 3 cups baby spinach
- 2 medium red onions, peeled, diced
- 2 1/2 cups tomatoes
- 3 cups cooked chickpeas
- 1 ½ teaspoon minced garlic
- 1/3 teaspoon ground black pepper
- 1 ¼ teaspoon salt
- 1/4 teaspoon allspice
- 1 tablespoon coconut sugar
- 1 teaspoon dried oregano
- 1/4 teaspoon cayenne
- 1/4 teaspoon cloves
- 2 bay leaves
- 1 tablespoon coconut oil

- 2 tablespoons olive oil
- 1 cup vegetable stock
- 1 lemon, juiced
- 2 ounces vegan feta cheese

Directions:

1. Take a large skillet pan, place it over medium-high heat, add coconut oil and when it melts, add onion and cook for 5 minutes until softened.
2. Switch heat to medium-low level, stir in garlic, cook for 2 minutes, then stir in tomatoes, add all the spices and bay leaves, pour in the stock, stir until mixed and cook for 20 minutes.
3. Then stir in chickpeas, simmer cooking for 15 minutes until the cooking liquid has reduced by one-third, stir in spinach and cook for 3 minutes until it begins to wilt.
4. Then stir in olive oil, sugar and lemon juice, taste to adjust seasoning, and remove and discard bay leaves.
5. When done, top chickpeas with cheese, broil for 5 minutes until cheese has melted and golden brown, then garnish with parsley and serve.

Sweet Potato and White Bean Skillet

Preparation time: 10 minutes

Cooking time: 45 minutes

Servings: 4

Ingredients:

- 1 large bunch of kale, chopped
- 2 large sweet potatoes, peeled,
- ¼-inch cubes
- 12 ounces cannellini beans
- 1 small onion, peeled, diced
- 1/8 teaspoon red pepper flakes
- 1 teaspoon salt
- 1 teaspoon cumin
- ½ teaspoon ground black pepper
- 1 teaspoon curry powder
- 1 1/2 tablespoons coconut oil
- 6 ounces coconut milk, unsweetened

Directions:

1. Take a large skillet pan, place it over medium heat, add ½ tablespoon oil and when it melts, add onion and cook for 5 minutes.

2. Then stir in sweet potatoes, stir well, cook for 5 minutes, then season with all the spices, cook for 1 minute and remove the pan from heat.

3. Take another pan, add remaining oil in it, place it over medium heat and when oil melts, add kale, season with some salt and black pepper, stir well, pour in the milk and cook for 15 minutes until tender.

4. Then add beans, beans, and red pepper, stir until mixed and cook for 5 minutes until hot.

5. Serve straight away.

Black Bean Burgers

Serves: 6 Time: 25 Minutes

Ingredients:

- 1 Onion, Diced
- ½ Cup Corn Nibs
- 2 Cloves Garlic, Minced
- ½ Teaspoon Oregano, Dried
- ½ Cup Flour
- 1 Jalapeno Pepper, Small
- 2 Cups Black Beans, Mashed & Canned
- ¼ Cup Breadcrumbs (Vegan)
- 2 Teaspoons Parsley, Minced
- ¼ Teaspoon Cumin
- 1 Tablespoon Olive Oil
- 2 Teaspoons Chili Powder
- ½ Red Pepper, Diced
- Sea Salt to Taste

Directions:

1. Set your flour on a plate, and then get out your garlic, onion, peppers and oregano, throwing it in a pan.
2. Cook over medium-high heat, and then cook until the onions are translucent.
3. Place the peppers in, and sauté until tender.
4. Cook for two minutes, and then set it to the side.
5. Use a potato masher to mash your black beans, and then stir in the vegetables, cumin, breadcrumbs, parsley, salt and chili powder, and then divide it into six patties.
6. Coat each side, and then cook until it's fried on each side.

Interesting Facts:

Potatoes are a great starchy source of potassium and protein. They are pretty inexpensive if you are one that is watching their budget. Bonus: Very heart-healthy!

Hearty Black Lentil Curry

Servings: 4

Preparation time: 6 hours and 35 minutes

Ingredients:

- 1 cup of black lentils, rinsed and soaked overnight
- 14 ounce of chopped tomatoes
- 2 large white onions, peeled and sliced
- 1 1/2 teaspoon of minced garlic
- 1 teaspoon of grated ginger
- 1 red chili
- 1 teaspoon of salt
- 1/4 teaspoon of red chili powder
- 1 teaspoon of paprika
- 1 teaspoon of ground turmeric
- 2 teaspoons of ground cumin
- 2 teaspoons of ground coriander
- 1/2 cup of chopped coriander
- 4-ounce of vegetarian butter
- 4 fluid of ounce water
- 2 fluid of ounce vegetarian double cream

Directions:

1. Place a large pan over an average heat, add butter and let heat until melt.
2. Add the onion along with garlic and ginger and let cook for 10 to 15 minutes or until onions are caramelized.
3. Then stir in salt, red chili powder, paprika, turmeric, cumin, ground coriander, and water.
4. Transfer this mixture to a 6-quarts slow cooker and add tomatoes and red chili.
5. Drain lentils, add to slow cooker and stir until just mix.
6. Plug in slow cooker; adjust cooking time to 6 hours and let cook on low heat setting.
7. When the lentils are done, stir in cream and adjust the seasoning.
8. Serve with boiled rice or whole wheat bread.

Smoky Red Beans and Rice

Servings: 6

Preparation time: 5 hours and 10 minutes

Ingredients:

- 30 ounce of cooked red beans
- 1 cup of brown rice, uncooked
- 1 cup of chopped green pepper
- 1 cup of chopped celery
- 1 cup of chopped white onion
- 1 1/2 teaspoon of minced garlic
- 1/2 teaspoon of salt
- 1/4 teaspoon of cayenne pepper
- 1 teaspoon of smoked paprika
- 2 teaspoons of dried thyme
- 1 bay leaf
- 2 1/3 cups of vegetable broth

Directions:

1. Using a 6-quarts slow cooker place all the ingredients except for the rice, salt and cayenne pepper.

67

2. Stir until it mixes properly and then cover the top.

3. Plug in the slow cooker; adjust the cooking time to 4 hours and let it steam on a low heat setting.

4. Then pour in and stir the rice, salt, cayenne pepper and continue cooking for an additional 2 hours at a high heat setting.

5. Serve straight away.

Creamy Artichoke Soup

Preparation time: 5 minutes

Cooking time: 40 minutes

Servings: 4

Ingredients:

- 1 can artichoke hearts, drained
- 3 cups vegetable broth
- 2 tbsp lemon juice
- 1 small onion, finely cut
- 2 cloves garlic, crushed
- 3 tbsp olive oil
- 2 tbsp flour
- ½ cup vegan cream

Directions:

1. Gently sauté the onion and garlic in some olive oil.
2. Add the flour, whisking constantly, and then add the hot vegetable broth slowly, while still whisking.
3. Cook for about 5 minutes.

4. Blend the artichoke, lemon juice, salt and pepper until smooth.

5. Add the puree to the broth mix, stir well, and then stir in the cream.

6. Cook until heated through.

7. Garnish with a swirl of vegan cream or a sliver of artichoke.

Super Rad-ish Avocado Salad

Preparation time: 10 minutes

Cooking time: 25 minutes

Servings: 2 Salads.

Ingredients:

- 6 shredded carrots
- 6 ounces diced radishes
- 1 diced avocado
- 1/3 cup ponzu

Directions:

1. Bring all the above ingredients together in a serving bowl and toss.
2. Enjoy!

Red Quinoa and Black Bean Soup

Preparation time: 5 minutes

Cooking time: 40 minutes 6 Servings.

Ingredients:

- 1 ¼ cup red quinoa
- 4 minced garlic cloves
- ½ tbsp.. coconut oil
- 1 diced jalapeno
- 3 cups diced onion
- 2 tsp. cumin
- 1 chopped sweet potato
- 1 tsp. coriander
- 1 tsp. chili powder
- 5 cups vegetable broth
- 15 ounces black beans
- ½ tsp. cayenne pepper
- 2 cups spinach

Directions:

1. Begin by bringing the quinoa into a saucepan to boil with two cups of water.
2. Allow the quinoa to simmer for twenty minutes.
3. Next, remove the quinoa from the heat.
4. To the side, heat the oil, the onion, and the garlic together in a large soup pot.
5. Add the jalapeno and the sweet potato and sauté for an additional seven minutes.
6. Next, add all the spices and the broth and bring the soup to a simmer for twenty-five minutes.
7. The potatoes should be soft.
8. Prior to serving, add the quinoa, the black beans, and the spinach to the mix.
9. Season, and serve warm. Enjoy.

Sunny Orange Carrot Soup

Preparation time: 5 minutes

Cooking time: 60 minutes 6 cups.

Ingredients:

- 2 tsp. coconut oil
- 2 cups diced onion
- 4 minced garlic cloves
- 1 cup orange juice
- 2 pounds chopped carrots
- 6 cups vegetable broth
- 3 tbsp. grated ginger
- 1 cup cashews
- salt and pepper to taste

Directions:

1. Begin by bringing the cashews into a bowl of water and allowing them to soak for one hour.
2. To the side, heat the oil, the onion, and the garlic together in a large soup pot.
3. Cook this mixture for three minutes.

4. Afterwards, add the orange juice, the carrots, the vegetable broth, and the ginger. S

5. tir well, and simmer to soup for twenty minutes.

6. Next, all the soup to cool for fifteen minutes.

7. To the side, drain the cashews and blend the cashews with the rest of the soup in a blender.

8. Next, pour the soup back in the soup pot, and test the seasonings.

9. Serve warm, and enjoy.

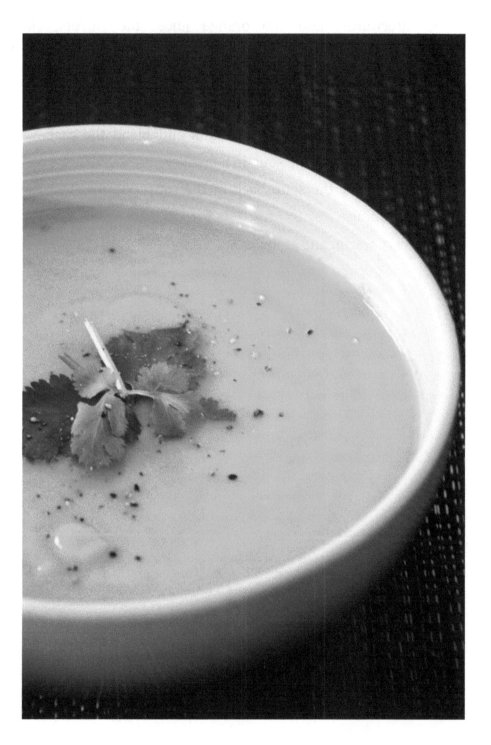

Broccoli Cheddar Vegan Soup

Preparation time: 5 minutes

Cooking time: 40 minutes 4 Servings.

Ingredients:

- 1 diced onion
- 1 tsp. olive oil
- 1 cup diced celery
- 3 minced garlic cloves
- 2 cups chopped potatoes
- 5 cups chopped broccoli
- 4 cups vegetable broth
- ½ tsp. cayenne pepper
- 2 tbsp. nutritional yeast
- 1 cup vegan cheese sauce
- salt and pepper to taste

Directions:

1. Begin by heating the onion, the garlic, and the oil together in a soup pot for about seven minutes.

2. Next, add the celery, the potatoes, and the broccoli to the pot.
3. Allow them to cook for six minutes.
4. Next, add the nutritional yeast, the broth, and the cayenne, and allow the soup to simmer for twenty minutes.
5. Next, pour the soup into a blender and blend the soup until it's nearly smooth.
6. Add the vegan cheese in between purees and mix well.
7. Next, pour the soup back in the soup pot and adjust salt and pepper seasoning.
8. Enjoy!

Chili Fennel

Preparation Time: 10 minutes

Cooking Time: 8 minutes

Ingredients

- 2 fennel bulbs, cut into quarters
- 3 tablespoons olive oil
- Salt and black pepper to the taste
- 1 garlic clove, minced
- 1 red chili pepper, chopped
- ¾ cup veggie stock Juice of
- ½ lemon

Directions:

1. Heat up a pan that fits your Air Fryer with the oil over medium-high heat, add garlic and chili pepper, stir and cook for 2 minutes.
2. Add fennel, salt, pepper, stock and lemon juice, toss to coat, introduce in your Air Fryer and cook at 350 ° F for 6 minutes.
3. Divide between plates and serve as a side dish.

Easy Mean White Bean Dip

Preparation time: 10 minutes

Cooking time: 30 minutes 10 servings.

Ingredients:

- 3 minced garlic cloves
- 16 ounces white beans
- 1 tbsp. olive oil
- 2 tbsp. lemon juice
- 1 tsp. salt
- ½ tsp. cumin
- 1 tsp. chili powder
- 3 drops hot pepper sauce

Directions:

1. Begin by placing all the ingredients together in a food processor, and process them for about two minutes or until they're smooth.
2. If your mixture is too thick and chunky, add water to the food processor until you reach your desired consistency.
3. Enjoy!

Roasted Red Pepper Soup

Preparation time: 5 minutes

Cooking time: 50 minutes

Servings: 5-6

Ingredients:

- 5-6 large red peppers
- 1 large onion, chopped
- 2 garlic cloves, crushed
- 4 medium tomatoes, chopped
- 4 cups vegetable broth
- 3 tbsp olive oil
- 2 bay leaves

Directions:

1. Grill the peppers or roast them in the oven at 400 F until the skins are a little burnt.
2. Place the roasted peppers in a brown paper bag or a lidded container and leave covered for about 10 minutes.
3. This makes it easier to peel them.
4. Peel the skins and remove the seeds.

5. Cut the peppers in small pieces.

6. Heat oil in a large saucepan over medium-high heat.

7. Add onion and garlic and sauté, stirring, for 3 minutes or until onion has softened.

8. Add the red peppers, bay leaves, tomato and simmer for 5 minutes.

9. Add broth.

10. Season with pepper.

11. Bring to the boil, then reduce heat and simmer for 20 more minutes.

12. Set aside to cool slightly.

13. Blend, in batches, until smooth and serve.

Quinoa, White Bean, and Kale Soup

Preparation time: 5 minutes

Cooking time: 60 minutes

Servings: 5-6

Ingredients:

- ½ cup uncooked quinoa, rinsed well
- 1 small onion, chopped
- 1 can diced tomatoes, undrained
- 2 cans cannellini beans, undrained
- 3 cups chopped kale
- 2 garlic cloves, chopped
- 4 cups vegetable broth
- 1 tsp paprika
- 1 tsp dried mint
- salt and pepper, to taste

Directions:

1. Combine all ingredients except the kale into the slow cooker.

2. Season with salt and pepper to taste.

3. Cook on high for 4 hours or low for 6-7 hours.

4. Add in kale about 30 minutes before soup is finished cooking.

Autumnal Apple and Squash Soup

Preparation time: 5 minutes

Cooking time: 60 minutes

6 Servings.

Ingredients:

- 2 pounds diced butternut squash
- 2 tbsp. olive oil
- 3 diced and peeled apples
- 32 ounces vegetable broth
- 3 tsp. ginger
- 1 diced onion
- 1 tsp. cumin
- 1 ½ tsp. curry powder
- 2 cups soymilk
- salt and pepper to taste

Directions:

1. Begin by preheating your oven to 375 degrees Fahrenheit.

2. Next, wrap the butternut squash with aluminum foil, and bake the squash for forty-five minutes.

3. Next, set them to the side to allow them to cool.

4. Afterwards, remove the seeds, and peel the skin off.

5. Slice and dice the squash.

6. Bring the squash and the soymilk together in a food processor, and pulse the ingredients.

7. Next, pour the oil into the bottom of the soup pot.

8. Add the onion and sauté the onion for five minutes.

9. Next, add the apple, the broth, and the spices.

10. Bring this mixture to a boil and then allow it to simmer on low for twelve minutes.

11. Next, puree this soup pot mixture in the blender or food processor, and place this back in the soup pot.

12. Add the squash and the soymilk to the mixture, and stir well.

13. Now, allow this soup to simmer for ten more minutes, and salt and pepper before serving.

14. Enjoy.

Spicy Vegetable Soup

Preparation time: 5 minutes

Cooking time: 20 minutes

6 Servings.

Ingredients:

- 1 cup soaked cashews
- 5 cups vegetable broth
- 3 diced garlic cloves
- 1 tbsp. olive oil
- 4 diced carrots
- 1 diced red pepper
- 2 chopped celery stalks
- 1 diced sweet potato
- 1 28-ounce can diced tomatoes
- 1 tsp. basil
- 1 tsp. paprika
- 1 tsp. cumin
- 2 cups spinach
- 15 ounce can of black beans

Directions:

1. Begin by soaking the cashews in a small bowl with water for two hours.
2. Next, bring the cashews and the vegetable broth together in a food processor.
3. Puree the mixture until it's smooth.
4. Next, heat the oil and the vegetables together for five minutes in a soup pot.
5. Add the spices, and stir, cooking for about seven minutes.
6. Next, add the vegetable broth, and continue to stir.
7. Allow the soup to simmer for twenty minutes.
8. Next, salt and pepper the mixture, and serve the soup warm.
9. Enjoy!

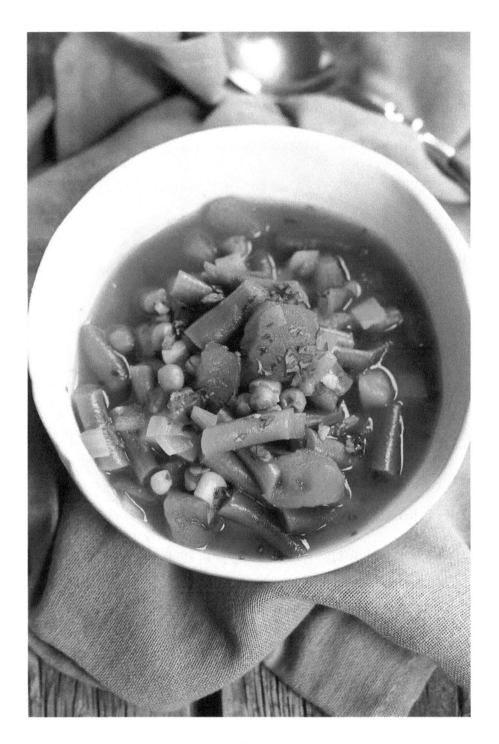

Bean and Carrot Spirals

Preparation time: 10 minutes

Cooking time: 40 minutes

24 servings.

Ingredients:

- 4 8-inch flour tortillas
- 1 ½ cups of Easy Mean White Bean dip (recipe found here)
- 10 ounces spinach leaves
- ½ cup diced carrots
- ½ cup diced red peppers

Directions:

1. Begin by preparing the bean dip, seen above.
2. Next, spread out the bean dip on each tortillas, making sure to leave about a ¾ inch white border on the outside of the tortillas.
3. Next, place spinach in the center of the tortilla, followed by carrots and red peppers.

4. Roll the tortillas into tight rolls, and then cover each of the rolls with plastic wrap or aluminum foil.

5. Allow them to chill in the fridge for twenty-four hours.

6. Afterwards, remove the wrap from the spirals and remove the very ends of the rolls.

7. Slice the rolls into six individual spiral pieces, and arrange them on a platter for serving.

8. Enjoy!

Very Vegan Crunchy Chile Nachos

Preparation time: 10 minutes

Cooking time: 50 minutes

8 Servings.

Ingredients:

- 14 corn tortillas.
- 1 minced onion
- 2 tsp. olive oil
- 1 diced tomato
- 1 diced garlic
- 1 tbsp. white flour
- 2 diced jalapeno peppers
- 4 tbsp. rice milk
- 7 ounce grated nondairy cheddar cheese

Directions:

1. Begin by preheating the oven to 375 degrees Fahrenheit.

2. Next, slice each of the corn tortillas into wedges and place them out on a baking sheet.

3. Allow them to bake for twenty minutes.

4. Afterwards, remove the chips and allow them to cool.

5. Heat garlic and onion together in some olive oil and sauté them for five minutes.

6. Afterwards, add the tomatoes and the jalapenos, and continue to cook and stir for one minute. Add the rice milk.

7. Next, pour the nondairy cheese into the mixture, and stir the ingredients together until the cheese completely melts.

8. Remove the skillet form the heat.

9. Spread out the tortillas on a large plate, and pour the created cheese sauce overtop the chips.

10. Serve warm.

Tofu Nuggets with Barbecue Glaze

9 Servings.

Ingredients:

- 32 ounces tofu
- 1 cup quick vegan barbecue sauce

Directions:

1. Begin by preheating the oven to 425 degrees Fahrenheit.
2. Next, slice the tofu and blot the tofu with clean towels.
3. Next, slice and dice the tofu and completely eliminate the water from the tofu material.
4. Stir the tofu with the vegan barbecue sauce, and place the tofu on a baking sheet.
5. Bake the tofu for fifteen minutes.
6. Afterwards, stir the tofu and bake the tofu for an additional ten minutes.
7. Enjoy!

Broiled Japanese Eggplants

Preparation time: 10 minutes

Cooking time: 50 minutes

4 Servings.

Ingredients:

- 2 tbsp. white wine
- 2 tbps. Sweet rice wine
- 3 tbsp. agave netar
- 4 tbsp. mellow white miso
- 4 Japanese eggplants, sliced in half, de-stemmed

Directions:

1. Begin by simmering the sweet rice wine and the white wine together in a saucepan.
2. Simmer them together for two minutes.
3. Afterwards, add the miso and stir the ingredients until they're smooth.
4. Add the agave nectar.
5. At this time, reduce the stovetop heat to low.

6. Continue to heat this mixture while you initiate the next step.
7. Next, place the eggplants with their cut-sides down onto the baking sheet.
8. Place the baking sheet in the broiler for three minutes.
9. Make sure that they do not burn.
10. After three minutes, flip them and cook them for an additional three minutes.
11. The tops should be brown.
12. After the eggplants have cooked, layer the created sauce overtop of them.
13. Place them in the broiler for about forty-five seconds.
14. Afterwards, remove the eggplants and serve them warm.
15. Enjoy!

Groovy Indian Samosas

Preparation time: 10 minutes

Cooking time: 30 minutes

4 Servings.

Ingredients:

- ¼ cup olive oil
- 2 diced onions
- 1 tsp. mustard seeds
- ½ tsp. salt
- 3 tsp. curry powder
- 1 diced carrot
- 2 diced potatoes
- 1 cup diced green beans
- 1 cup frozen peas
- 1/3 cup water
- 8 ounces phyllo pastry sunflower or olive oil for frying

Directions:

1. Begin by warming up the olive oil in a skillet, and adding the mustard seeds, allowing them to heat until they pop.
2. Add the onions, and cook them for five minutes.
3. Next, pour in the curry powder and the salt.
4. Fry these together for one and a half minutes.
5. Next, add the carrots, the potatoes, the peas, the beans, and the water.
6. Cook this mixture together for fifteen minutes on LOW.
7. The vegetables should be soft.
8. Next, slice up the phyllo pastry to create long strips.
9. Take one strip and place a tbsp.. of the created filling in the strip, at the end.
10. Fold this strip diagonally to create a triangle.
11. Continue this folding until the very end of the strip.
12. Afterwards, seal up the end with water.
13. Repeat the above steps with all the remaining phyllo strips.
14. Afterwards, half-fill a wok with sunflower oil.
15. Heat the oil to 350 degrees Fahrenheit.
16. Next, fry up the samosas for three minutes until they reach a golden color.
17. Allow them to drain, and then serve them warm.
18. Enjoy!

Vegan Creation Coleslaw

Preparation time: 10 minutes

Cooking time: 30 minutes

3 cups.

Ingredients:

- 1 cup cashews
- 2 tbsp. agave syrup
- juice of 2 lemons
- 1 tsp. mustard
- 1 tsp. Dijon mustard
- 1/3 cup sliced almonds
- 1/3 cup shredded cabbage
- 3 cups shredded spinach
- 4 springs parsley

Directions:

1. Begin by adding cashews, agave, and lemon juice together in a food processor.
2. Process well, and add the mustards.

3. Next, mix together the almonds, the spinach, the cabbage, and the parsley.
4. Add the sauce to the mixture, and serve.
5. Enjoy!

Finger-Licking Appetizer Pretzels

Preparation time: 10 minutes

 Cooking time: 40 minutes

5 cups.

Ingredients:

- 3 cups small pretzels
- 3 tbsp. soy sauce
- 1 tsp. cinnamon
- 3 tbsp. agave nectar
- 2 cups unsalted peanuts or almonds
- ½ tsp. ginger

Directions:

1. Begin by preheating the oven to 300 degrees Fahrenheit.
2. Next, bring together the soy sauce, the cinnamon, the agave nectar, and the ginger in a medium-sized bowl.
3. Stir well.

4. Add the pretzels and the nuts and continue to stir.

5. Spread this creation over a baking sheet, and bake them for twenty minutes.

6. You should stir them every five minutes.

7. Next, allow the pretzels to cool, and set them out as a party appetizer.

8. Enjoy!

Appetizing Cucumber Salad

Preparation time: 20 minutes

Cooking time: 0 minutes

Servings: 4

Ingredients:

- 2 cucumber, peeled
- 3 tablespoons olive oil
- 1 cup sour cream
- 1 tbsp fresh lemon juice
- 1 garlic clove, peeled and minced
- 1/3 cup fresh dill leaves, chopped roughly

What you'll need from the store cupboard:

- ½ tsp pepper
- Salt to taste

Directions:

1. Slice cucumber into 3 equal lengths.
2. Then slice lengthwise into quarters or smaller to create cucumber sticks.

3. Drain in a colander and set aside.

4. In a medium bowl whisk well the remaining ingredients.

5. Add the drained cucumber into a bowl of dressing and toss well to coat.

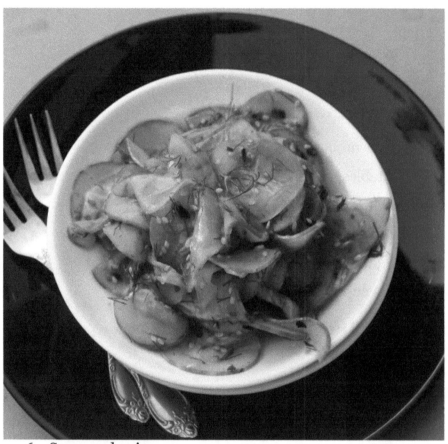

6. Serve and enjoy.

Long Beans Mix

Preparation Time: 10 minutes

Cooking Time: 10 minutes

Ingredients

- ½ teaspoon coconut aminos
- 1 tablespoon olive oil
- A pinch of salt and black pepper
- 4 garlic cloves, minced
- 4 long beans, trimmed and sliced

Directions:

1. In a pan that fits your Air Fryer, combine long beans with oil, aminos, salt, pepper and garlic, toss, introduce in your Air Fryer and cook at 350° F for 10 minutes.
2. Divide between plates and serve as a side dish.

Scalloped Potatoes

Preparation Time: 10 minutes

Cooking time: 4 hours

Servings: 8

Ingredients:

- Cooking spray
- 2 pounds gold potatoes, halved and sliced
- 1 yellow onion, cut into medium wedges
- 10 ounces canned vegan potato cream soup
- 8 ounces coconut milk
- 1 cup tofu, crumbled
- ½ cup veggie stock
- Salt and black pepper to the taste
- 1 tablespoons parsley, chopped

Directions:

1. Coat your slow cooker with cooking spray and arrange half of the potatoes on the bottom.
2. Layer onion wedges, half of the vegan cream soup, coconut milk, tofu, stock, salt and pepper.

3. Add the rest of the potatoes, onion wedges, cream, coconut milk, tofu and stock, cover and cook on High for 4 hours.

4. Sprinkle parsley on top, divide scalloped potatoes between plates and serve as a side dish.

5. Enjoy!

Cauliflower and Broccoli Side Dish

Preparation Time: 10 minutes

Cooking time: 3 hours

Servings: 10

Ingredients:

- 4 cups broccoli florets
- 4 cups cauliflower florets
- 14 ounces tomato paste
- 1 yellow onion, chopped
- 1 teaspoon thyme, dried
- Salt and black pepper to the taste
- ½ cup almonds, sliced

Directions:

1. In your slow cooker, mix broccoli with cauliflower, tomato paste, onion, thyme, salt and pepper, toss, cover and cook on High for 3 hours.

2. Add almonds, toss, divide between plates and serve as a side dish.
3. Enjoy!

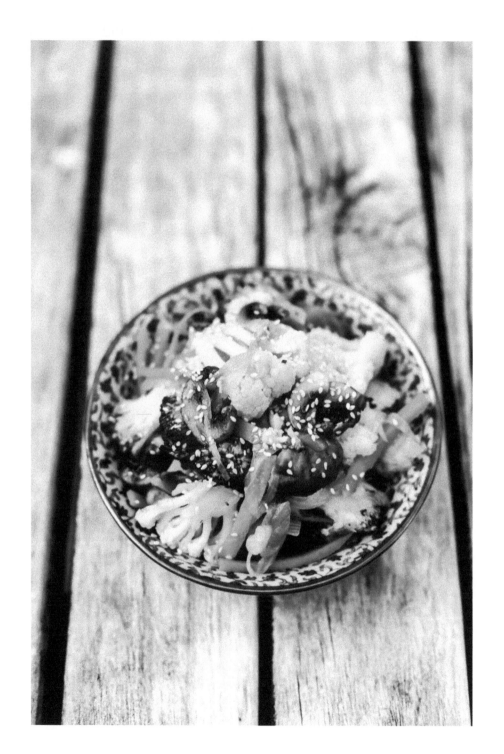